The HCG Diet:

Lose Weight Quickly and Safely for Life with the HCG Diet Plan

BENJAMIN TIDEAS

.

CONTENTS

INTRODUCTION

I want to thank you and congratulate you for grabbing this book, "The HCG Diet: Lose Weight Quickly and Safely for Life with the HCG Diet Plan".

This book contains proven steps and strategies on how to finally lose the weight you've wanted with the HCG Diet. More importantly, this book also focuses on keeping that weight off for good. There are obviously many diet plans available to anyone wanting to shed those extra pounds. If you are to try the hCG Diet, the significant questions that arise are:

- Is it safe?
- Does it produce rapid results?
- Will it provide lasting results?
- Is it right for your plan and your lifestyle?

This book aims to answer the questions mentioned above, give you specifics, arm you with resources and show you just how effectively the HCG diet can work for you.

Thanks again for picking up this book, I hope you enjoy it!

Also, Don't forget to grab your FREE Bonuses via the link at the end!

Now, let's get to it!

FUNDAMENTALS OF THE HCG DIET

What is the hCG Diet?

The hCG Diet is the meal component of the hCG weight loss protocol. The protocol was designed by Dr. Albert T. W. Simeons, a British endocrinologist, who devoted his professional life to searching for remedies to health conditions and solutions to medical paradoxes that bring suffering to humanity. The diet component consists of a 550 to 800 calories (cal) meal program. In addition to a calorie-restricted diet, the weight-loss protocol also includes regular hCG injections and regular exercise components.

The hCG in the hCG diet stands for human chorionic gonadotropin, a hormone that alters the female reproductive environment during pregnancy. Its function is to convert the stored body fat of the pregnant woman into nutrition for the developing baby. In this book, the abbreviation for the hormone may be expressed interchangeably in its standard medical acronym with the small letter "h" or the upper-case initials HCG. The hCG hormone is secreted by the syncytiotrophoblast, which is found in the fertilized egg after conception. For those who know well about female reproductive anatomy, the term "chorionic" forms part of the hormone's name because it is produced in the chorion layer of the placenta. Meanwhile, the term "gonadotropin" completes the hormone name; because during pregnancy, hCG drives the corpus luteum (a yellowish structure performing some endocrine functions during pregnancy). It is similar to what the luteinizing hormone from the pituitary gland does during normal female reproductive cycles.

From years of assisting obese and overweight patients with the hCG program, some modifications to the initial protocol have been made to attune the program to the patients' condition. The changes produced better, safer, and longer-lasting results. Basically, the current hCG diet consists of some fixes like taking 550 and 800 calories a day. The breakfast consists of protein and fruit serving. Additional fruit serving and protein accompanied by more green vegetables. Take multi-vitamins and mineral prescribed by physician. Patient's medication can be taken. hCG administration that may be given as an intravenous injection, as a sub-cutaneous injection, or orally in sublingual form is required. Find out the protocol related products that are readily available.

With the enhancements to the original hCG diet's restricted daily calorie intake range, the popular weight loss program was found to be more tolerable to patients. It was also much safer but produced similar results as the previous 500 cal daily restriction. In addition, with a slightly increased calorie limit per day, those who are subscribed to the protocol are more successful in completing the program, as they have fewer complaints of headache, hunger, and weakness.

Benefits of the hCG Diet

The enhanced hCG diet with slightly increased calorie limit obtained mostly from additional sources of protein offers multiple benefits. First of all, it assists the body in preserving the lean muscle mass. It also increases the burning of stored fat. Fantastically it curbs appetite as much as 40% throughout the day.

In addition to the increased meal protein content, the hCG has other benefits to offer. It enhances body metabolism. While dieting, fat burning is achieved without causing lean muscle wasting. It minimizes attraction for sweet consumption Another remarkable thing is, it creates the feeling of natural fullness that is indeed necessary to dieting without starving. As a result of fat distribution, flabbiness decreases.

Beginnings and Development of the hCG Diet

Dr. Simeons' passion, for treating the ills suffered by mankind, was no secret as he pioneered on a drug against malaria and conducted research on the bubonic plague as well as on leprosy in India. In the 1950s, he shifted his investigations on the growing cases of obesity and a corresponding weight-loss intervention. Dr. Simeons also made research on the hCG hormone.

Accordingly, the hormone is extracted from the urine of pregnant women. The hCG was then used as an intervention for young boys afflicted with Froelich Syndrome. The disorder, which manifests as endocrine abnormalities, mostly affects young boys who appear obese, have oversized breasts and have undersized genitals. Treating these boys with hCG injections made them lose their big appetites and reduced their hip measurements as they began losing their belly fat.

A woman who sought his medical assistance for weight loss consultation became the impetus for his now historic breakthrough in a no-nonsense weight reduction program mainly through a specially designed diet and hCG injections. The woman was emaciated or abnormally thin as Dr. Simeons surveyed her top half visually while seated at his table as he talks on the phone. The lower half of his patient's body was obscured from his sight.

The patient had dry, loose skin with her ribs and collarbones protruding and she wanted to lose weight. The woman politely volunteered the information that she is not mad or crazy about the intent of her consultation. The woman rounded the doctor's desk revealing her lower half with large hips and thighs that do not necessarily complement her small waist. But what she is yet to know: she may be seeing the wrong doctor.

Dr. Simeons treated the top-emaciated and bottom-flabby woman with 125 IU (a pharmacological abbreviation which stands for international units); he also administered through daily intravenous (IV) injections. It combined with a calorie restricted diet and 30 minutes of daily walking. The treatment lasted eight weeks and the woman lost an average of one inch each week around her hips. Additionally, the woman was able to discard her fat reserves.

Success of the diet was not, however, a one-shot deal. Initial success with the lady patient was followed by a decade of hard work developing the protocol. Accordingly, Dr. Simeons experimented with specific dosages of hCG and specific food combinations to optimize weight loss faster but did away with the fat on a more permanent basis.

Dr. Simeons' diligent work with the hCG diet appealed to both embattled obesity patients and those who only care about managing their weight. By 1967, his clinic in Rome attracted diet subscribers in droves. His weight loss and weight management protocol sparked even the interest of Hollywood celebrities who are afraid of the flab. His hCG diet became the toast of Hollywood, the rich and famous, and not to mention royalty.

His weight loss protocol stirred even other members of the medical community that other doctors come to learn from him. At about this time, Dr. Simeons compiled his vast knowledge of the hCG diet and the weight loss protocol in his book, which he aptly called "Pounds and Inches: A New Approach to Obesity." However, even with its huge success and popularity, the hCG diet underwent setbacks not in the therapy and results, but in terms of government regulation and negative criticisms.

hCG as a drug was approved in 1970 by the Federal Drug Administration only as a medication to enhance fertility. In 1976, Dr. Simeons was compelled by the Federal Trade Commission to use a disclaimer about the FDA approval. The reason was to pronounce its efficacy as a treatment for obesity, as well as the vaunted attractive fat redistribution effect and the inconvenience of the diet's very low-calorie intake.

Some complaints of patient discomforts and criticisms regarding the lack of clinical studies, a modification of the hCG diet was implemented, and clinical studies were undertaken. It was a response to the criticisms about the starvation technically resulting from the limited calorie intake. A summary is presented in the last chapter, and complaints of patient discomfort ceased.

The hCG diet regimen is now better, safer, and more comfortable than ever. With time, it stood the test and has produced scientific evidence of its claim as a weight-loss protocol. Thus evolved the colorful events in the history of the hCG diet.

CLINICAL STUDIES: SCIENTIFIC BASIS OF THE HCG DIET

Despite the success of the original 500 calorie hCG diet, traditional medicine criticized the protocol about its safety because 500 cal is technically starving patients. On the side of diet subscribers were complaints about fatigue, headaches, hunger, and weakness. These are just the first two primary reasons why modifications were in order for the sake of patients who need to lose weight. What they wanted was getting back the pounds and inches they lost, but are unsure if they wish to try the hCG diet.

A clinical study on patients who were administered hCG with the modified diet lost an average of 19.84 pounds within a span of 6 weeks compared to the 14.75 pounds average loss of patients who had meals without hCG. The average decrease in BMI of the two groups of patients was also significant at 3.18 vs. 2.48, respectively.

American Journal of Clinical Nutrition showed that patients on the 500 calorie diet plus hCG did not complain of weakness or hunger. It came at a time when the complaints aired by some of the patients with the original 500 calorie diet. These patients reported having felt anywhere from good to excellent. The hCG group lost more weight on the average than the group on placebo.

PHASE 1: THE PRE-DIETING OR CLEANSING PHASE

The original formulation of the hCG diet, as designed by its creator Dr. Simeons, organized the protocol into three Phases. However, other trained practitioners of the hCG weight loss program added a fourth Phase. This chapter discusses the program as it is today, but will include information about the changes from the original Simeons design.

However practitioners call this Phase (pre-dieting cleansing or detox Phase), it all boils down to one thing: this is not the diet proper, but a preparatory stage for losing weight. In essence, this Phase would be a total body and colon cleanse as well as Candida yeast cleanse. The cleansing Phase takes two weeks, one month, or one and a half months.

This cleansing Phase is necessary not just for the hCG diet, but for any other weight loss regimen. The cleansing Phase is important because many food items today include substances that should not be part of a healthy diet. It is not just junk food and a ton of cholesterol that is being referred to here, but also a lot of toxins you wouldn't even be aware you ingested. Or you didn't know that it may not be alright for people about to embark on weight management-related dieting. Phase 1 of the hCG diet aims to expel the following toxins out of your body:

- Artificial flavorings such as brominated vegetable oils
- Antibiotics
- Artificial coloring or dyes in food
- Carcinogens coming from cooking at very high temperature, like acrylamide, heterocyclic amines, polycyclic aromatic hydrocarbons

7

- Dangerous chemicals from food processing such as potassium aluminum sulfate, sodium aluminum sulfate, and sodium nitrate or nitrite
- Dangerous chemicals from food packaging such as bisphenol-A
- Dioxins from fatty foods
- Genetically modified organism
- Growth hormones (in the meat you eat)
- Flavor Enhancers
- Herbicides
- Pesticides

You do not want the products mentioned above hanging around your gastrointestinal (GI) tract. Not that they have not yet done much damage, but cleansing will prevent these toxins from sticking to your GI system and cause further harm to your health and your weight loss/management goal. You don't want these toxins to clog your bowels for two reasons: Toxins in the GI tract will compromise your body's ability to absorb nutrients; Toxin-laced or toxin-clogged GI will also slow down your weight loss.

Meanwhile, a Candida yeast cleanse may proceed before or after the diet. Aside from toxins, build-up of Candida yeast over time may also prevent you from losing weight. In addition, it will also weaken the body's immune system and cause your metabolism to slow down. If the Candida yeast cleanse is to be made before the diet proper, Phase 1 will last one month if you opt for the 15-day yeast cleanse. However, should you go for the 30-day Candida yeast cleanse, Phase 1 will take one and a half months. The two cleansing procedures cannot be done simultaneously, and the yeast cleanse should precede the total body cleanse.

If a diet subscriber prefers to have the Candida cleanse after the diet proper, Phase 1 lasts only for two weeks. The yeast cleanse can be undertaken at Phase 3 or Phase 4. The yeast cleanse cannot be made during the diet proper or Phase 2.

General guidelines for Phase 1

As you start this Phase, you need a multi-vitamin and mineral supplement to sustain your low-calorie diet when you reach Phase 2 and to provide every tissue and organ of your body with essential nutrients.

Talk to your physician to know if it is safe for you to take a coral calcium supplement, as well as the correct dosage.

If you are taking any prescribed medication prior to your subscription to the hCG program, you are allowed to take them. The modified protocol allows medications, unlike the original plan formulation where a patient needed to stop all medications while subscribed to the hCG diet. However, if you have such medications, clear first with your personal physician if the other supplements are not contraindicated, although hCG supplements are usually fine with other medications.

Safely expose yourself to the sun; 10 to 15 minutes of early morning sun is recommended.

Since water is a natural cleanser, drink at least half a gallon of filtered water which may be combined with herbal tea with no sugar. Walk for at least 30 minutes daily or alternately, you can perform light physical activities for the same amount of time that may include Biking, Pilates, Swimming or Yoga.

Perform natural colon cleansing by avoiding laxatives, cleansers kits, and enema. Instead, eat the following natural colon cleansing foods based on a modified food pyramid: At least ten servings of fruits and vegetables daily making them the base of your cleansing food pyramid. These can include Apples (or raw Bragg apple cider vinegar), Avocadoes, Grapefruit (a potent body fat releaser), Lemons or Oranges.

Whole grain cereals and non-wheat or non-bread whole grains will take the place of fruits and vegetables in the food pyramid. By time, they will be reduced to only 2 to 4 servings, such as Amaranth, Barley, Buckwheat, Brown Rice, Millet, Oats, Quinoa, Rye or Spelt.

Protein foods, which retain their place in the food pyramid, with 4 to 6 servings, such as Beans, Eggs, Fish, Meat or Poultry. Flax seeds are great cleansers of the colon. Bragg apple cider vinegar may be used in salads, as a marinade, or as a substitute for cooking oil. Like grapefruit, it helps expel fat. If you need sugar in some of your foods, use a natural sweetener and avoid artificial sweeteners (e.g. Equal, Splenda).

Another change in the formulation of the hCG diet is to eat a healthy breakfast. Eating a healthy breakfast helps in burning fat, enhances metabolism, and provides energy by increasing your blood sugar. Ensure the recommended serving of the food groups in the modified pyramid into 5 parts. Smaller but more frequent meals are healthier than bigger meals, hasten your metabolism and help in releasing your body's stored fat. Consume fresh vegetable salad as a snack to provide fiber for blood sugar regulation and to stimulate digestion.

When shopping for food, select organic products, or if these are not available, always try observing some fixed shopping tips. For example, look for chicken that are not exposed to antibiotics. Eat fishes that are only caught from natural sources. Buy vegetables and fruits that were not exposed to pesticides.

In addition to fiber from food, a fiber supplement can help relieve any constipation and reduce appetite in addition to improving both digestion and metabolism. Use colon cleanse and Candida yeast cleanse supplements.

Don't make the mistake of only replacing regular soda with diet or no-sugar soda. Eliminate all carbonated drinks from your cleansing menu.

What to Avoid While on a Colon Cleanse

Complex carbohydrates are to be avoided throughout the hCG program. They are found in Bread, Cereal, Granola bars, Legumes, Nuts, Oatmeal, Pasta, Potatoes, Rice (refined, white), Canned Food, Dairy products. Also included are Fast food, fried food, Monosodium glutamate (MSG), Products with high fructose corn syrup (a culprit in the obesity epidemic and blood sugar level spikes that trigger diabetes) and other Sweets.

PHASE 2: THE DIET PLUS HCG INJECTION (OR DROPS) PHASE

Phase 2 is the hCG diet proper and the best way to introduce the nagging question being asked about the hCG protocol: Will people lose the same amount of weight if they opt not to take the injections? Well, once and for all, the answer is either yes or quite maybe. Each person is a special case, and if the diet alone offered good results to one, it might not be so for another. One factor is individual differences, and there are many other factors involved, like adherence to the diet and endocrine or hypothalamus conditions of the diet subscriber. A clinical study revealed that those who used hCG with the modified diet lost more weight than those who did not.

However, hCG is not just the terminology. It is a significant part of the weight-loss regimen, and that is the reason the protocol was named hCG diet. Dr. Simeons, other hCG diet experts, and this author are one in the consensus that the diet alone can make you lose the same amount of weight as another person who was not taking the natural way.

If you want truly lasting results, the diet alone cannot make false promises. It is the hCG that will prevent you from having food binges. Because you are too-lazy-to-exercise days and because, you are too hungry to fight your urge to eat and too weak to have the willpower to walk or do any other exercises. You need the hCG injections or the hCG drops to sustain you in this protocol. As a result, you will not complain or experience the disturbing conditions brought about by low-calorie diet such as having increasing hunger as the program progresses. Feeling lack of energy all the time and sometimes headaches might follow that. The lean muscles may be wasting. And most of all: a super-slow metabolism.

The following is a walk-through of how you will go about Phase 2:

Days 1-2: Loading Days: You weigh yourself without clothes right after you have woken up and emptied your bladder (i. e. urination). Record your weight on your tracking sheet.

Take the hCG as directed [Note: Doing this at home is easier with hCG drops, but if you prefer injections, follow the directions on your kit to the letter. You can always manage to do the injections yourself with the subcutaneous injections. Let a nurse or an hCG diet clinical specialist administer the intravenous injections if this will be your option.]

Eat fats and complex carbohydrates ONLY ON LOADING DAYS 1 AND 2. This prepares you for the subsequent low-calorie diet. Indulge in your favorite foods because you need them for reserve fats during the rest of Phase 2.

A minimum of 1/2 gallon of filtered water ought to be consumed in one day.

Day 3-40: You weigh yourself without clothes right after you have woken up and emptied your bladder (i.e. urination). Record your weight on your tracking sheet.

Administer the hCG as directed. Drink half a gallon to one full gallon of filtered water or bottled water throughout the day.

Eat meals based on the food guide and refrain from skipping meals. Your calorie intake must be in the range 550 to 799 cal and never exceed 800 cal.

Day 41-43: Stop the hCG administration. Continue with the Phase 2 diet plan as in days 3 to 40.

Take the following supplements for Phase 2 to sustain your low-calorie diet:

- Essential fatty acids in the form of Omega 3 and 6
- Fat burners, particularly calcium pyruvate
- Multivitamins and minerals whole food supplement

Here is a general guideline for phase 2 for your daily meal

servings. It is recommended to have 3 fruits a day, however, for people who've got insulin resistance it is required to consult with the physical first. Egg whites are counted as 1 protein; consuming 3 such servings is required. Also, take two servings of vegetables rich in fiber. And, eat a serving of salad.

The following are essential for diet subscribers under Phase two and it is recommended that they have these on hand:

- Accurate weighing scale (for your body weight)
- All natural sea salt (or Pink Himalayan)
- Bragg apple cider vinegar (organic)
- Food scale
- Garlic-pepper grinder
- George Foreman Grill
- Stevia (natural sweetener)

PHASE 3: THE STABILIZATION PHASE

This is the most critical Phase of the hCG protocol because your efforts and success in this Phase will help shape long-lasting results. Your goal in Phase 3 is to reset your body's rate of metabolism and stabilize or maintain your weight to within 2 pounds of your weight when you ended the second Phase. This takes 3 weeks, and the good news is: NO MORE INJECTIONS. Make sure you do not go on a food binge so that you won't need to do the protocol all over again; it's all up to you! The secret of weight loss is not wasting all your triumphs in losing your excess pounds only to get them back after the program by overeating and overindulging in food. You will now go beyond 800 cal daily, but pace yourself for your sake.

So, here is the complete guideline for phase three: It follows from phase 2 where we left it. Continue with low-calorie diet for 72 hours at least and then get started with the phase 3. As usual, keep breakfast. Also, weighing should be continued as dictated by phase 2. Increase the amount of vegetables and fruits intake. You can take six meals a day on top. It is necessary to increase the number of protein servings. Always avoid sugars and starches!

To make things very clear, the danger foods in Phase 3 are the following and under no circumstances should you eat them: Bread, Pastries, Potatoes, Rice, Sugar (of course!)

You can eat practically anything but follow all the Phase 4 guidelines (next).

PHASE 4: THE MAINTENANCE PHASE

Phase 4, the maintenance stage of the protocol, begins after three weeks of the stabilization Phase or after you have kept a consistent weight within 2 pounds. Some subscribers to the diet may not need Phase 4 in order to reintroduce sugars and starches (i. e. those who have diabetes and those who have developed insulin resistance). However, all dieters need this Phase to stay focused on their lifelong goal which is to maintain the results of the weight loss program on a lasting basis. The best guide for this Phase is to start slow on your sugar and starches. Never go bingeing.

You may have missed the chocolates, and you may have half a bar this week and some another day in the other weeks. If you love bread, do not consume it together with chocolate; wait for several days. This is what is meant by starting slowly and safely to avoid getting back the lost pounds in a jiffy. Phase 4 will have the longest duration—the rest of your life.

You have to observe how your body reacts to the sugars and starches that you have discarded for a long time. As you do this, stay focused and motivated by keeping the right mindset. Do not think, "I ought to stay within 140 pounds, my ideal weight for my friends to notice." This is considered limiting language. Instead, you say, "I want to keep my 140 pound ideal weight for good health."

If you want to keep your ideal weight, then take care in maintaining it. Never let go of your maintenance efforts. You do not wish to lose more weight than is necessary or regain the weight you lost through the protocol.

Another thing, keep your weight tracking sheet during the regimen and for the rest of your life. The rationale is two-fold: You need a sheet to monitor and record weight gain or loss and you need a written way to stay focused on your goal.

Besides your tracking sheet, keep your body measurements which will inspire you to eat healthily and expel the pounds you don't need just by looking at the inches you lost. Typical measurements will be Shoulders, Chest, Waist, Biceps, Abdomen, Hips Thighs and Calves.

Just remember, if you are gaining weight - look back on what sugar, starch or fatty foods you had and decrease your intake. Or better yet, stop eating that food item for a while and see what happens. It's a good practice to keep a food log. It is always easy to see where you went overboard just by looking at the log. My favorite online version is myfitnesspal.com. The rest is up to you!

STAYING MOTIVATED WHILE DIETING

Of all the challenges that come up with dieting, staying motivated is the most difficult one. Often times while dieting, you will find yourself in a position where it's so hard to cope with the everyday struggle of dieting. Let alone the temptations that allure you each moment, which are really hard to resist. But remember that you are not the only person on the planet to be going through this hurdle, there are many like you who are trying day and night and many who have succeeded.

Instead of dieting, consider it eating healthy

Remind yourself all the time: by dieting you have opened up a new door to your lifestyle; on the other side of that awaits a healthy and happy lifestyle. The only purpose of dieting is not weight loss. Living a healthy and revived life is what should be considered as the primary goal of dieting in the first place. When you are feeling a lot better than before, physically, it boosts your mental ability as well, which will be reflected in a boosted confidence level. Consider it a transition from one eating habit to another, eating better every day rather than eating random foods every day. Aren't you feeling a little better already?

Set up credible, attainable goals

Dieting is not an overnight process. If you are considering losing few pounds within days and dreaming of a modeling figure, then you couldn't be more wrong. Instead of thinking of crossing the hurdle with a long jump, establish month wise goals and enter them in your diet calendar. Take one step at a time. As your body metabolism becomes used to a reduced or controlled diet, the task becomes so easy. And, of course, a Quantum scale can be preferable to a regular scale found in the market. A Quantum scale will show the progress converted in numbers. Thus, it should help you to get rid of any kind of frustration or bad feelings.

Get Rewarded

Rewarding is a great part of any motivation program, whether it's a dog training program or teaching a toddler. So why don't apply it in your case as well? With positive reinforcement, you will feel motivated and try retaining the positive attitude throughout your weight loss journey. Suppose – you have been avoiding delicious dark chocolates for a month or two, then you may like to spend it on something valuable like a gadget or ornaments. With this reward, you are incessantly reminding yourself of the sacrifices you are making and its return. Just be mindful, not to ambush your progress with a reward of something you shouldn't eat. My favorite rewards are things that will also help in my goals. Perhaps, next time you reach a body fat percentage milestone, you get yourself a new smart scale or a better heart rate monitor. Be creative and make it fun, just don't make it chocolate!

Cut the amount of sweet intake, but not totally!

Giving up something for once and all can be really tough on you, especially, when you have been consuming it for a long time. This may lead to great amount of frustration. The best idea is to limit and to constrain the demand rather than quitting it totally. It's not a grave sin if you take a piece of chocolate now and then. It's alright as long as you are following the rules towards staying in shape.

Find all the positives in your life

Now that you are aiming to stay motivated, you can enjoy every moment of your life to its fullest. Do a little barnstorming to understand what makes you happy. It might be that you were thinking of establishing your own book club, or you were thinking of joining the tennis training sessions, or else what about attending cooking classes? Because of your health you may not have been having the courage to do this in the past; but now that you are changing this is the best time to make them happen. Who knows these social congregations might be a great opportunity for you to meet new people who are going through the same phase as yours?

The good thing about losing some weight is that as you start losing some points, your confidence level goes up. Consider replacing your wardrobe with new fashionable, smaller clothes—this should be a great boost for your cause. Take others' compliments with a thankful manner, and often, encourage yourself about the progress made so far. The ability to encourage oneself is a unique quality of persons who believe themselves, people who're strong and stay firm toward their goal in life.

Take it slow

Whatever you are planning to do, let it be slow. Don't be hasty, or, otherwise the chances are good that you will stumble. The weight loss trend will remain intact as you achieve with slowly and gradually. Don't follow people who believe by starving they are getting thin very fast—the truth is eventually one way or another they fail. According to nutritionists, skipping 200 calories a day is not even felt, when you are doing it on a daily basis. You must be enthusiastic to know that optimum weight loss is just one or two pounds a week!

Don't be afraid of setbacks

There is no doubt that temptations will always be surrounding you in the form of a hot fudge sundae or stacked cheeseburgers. There is no harm if you take a little bit sometimes. But the real problem is when you can't control yourself, thinking, "what's wrong if I eat the whole thing this time only?" In doing so, you are following a dangerous path, and as a result of that you can erase all of your progress.

Forget Perfectionism

Think of a situation when accidently you have eaten a full pint of ice cream before noon. When you are dieting such an incident is not so uncommon, but it doesn't necessarily mean that you have lost everything just because now there is a stain on your 'perfect' record. Don't give up, don't even think of it. Now you have indulged in 1000 calories accidently, but after that, you would not hesitate to consume 1000 calories a day. If you get back on track, your body will be none the wiser a week from now. If you stumble, just regroup and move forward as correctly as you can. Your past does not equal your future.

The Buddy System

Making a life change alone can be quite daunting. When you know other people who are up to the same cause as yours, it makes it a lot easier. There are times when we feel we can't do it, it's impossible for us. During that bumpy stage, your comrades in arms may come as a helping hand you to show you that the road is not bad as it seems. Time to time they are expected to share their ideas with you and keep you encouraged. You may also find inspiration from someone's different way of doing it. Humans are social animals, and keeping each other inspired and encouraged are some of the best methods to success you can aspire to.

SETTING EFFECTIVE AND ATTAINABLE WEIGHT LOSS GOALS

Have you set up the points that will be part of your weight-loss goal? If so, you have a clear understanding of the way ahead. Your next move has to be, detecting the short and long steps toward being able to proceed. It ought to be followed by the steps that are feasible and applicable right from this moment.

Effective goal setting plays the most vital role in implementing any weight-loss program. It is the foundation of all that will follow next. Lots of research has been done on this topic so far. However, here we have tried to show the pinpoints toward setting effective and attainable weight loss goals. Again be advised: there is much of this info on the web or anywhere else, but we've only decided to get started with the gist. Indeed, these 6 steps are the cornerstone of all others.

1. Challenging

With every weight loss ambition there comes a lot of difficulties. It also takes you to set up some challenges from your side too. So be sure of your capabilities before taking challenges. Don't make it so hard by being burdened with challenges that are very hard to realize—in this way, you would be wasting your time and motivation. Yesterday you may have been a couch potato having all kinds of pungent foods containing cholesterol and carbohydrates. But today, you are trying to be the world's fittest athlete. This is indeed not possible or feasible. So the goals have to be set up in a way that they will bear long term importance as well as they won't get boring or so hard to implement.

For example, you can always start with drinking 8 cups of water daily; however, this won't solely cut the fat you are willing to lose. So, make a reason for drinking, like doing cardio or other sweaty exercise and drink all the water you need afterward.

2. Attainable

Challenges are good as long as you don't cross the limit. At first try understanding what you can and cannot do. Only after being fully sure of yourself, you can set up attainable goals. If you fail to do it, you may feel frustrated from the moment you start your weight loss journey.

Example: No doubt extended aerobic exercise is well enough for your physical and mental well-being. Yesterday you exercised for 30 minutes and today you are aiming for 60 minutes—absolutely that's an improvement. But don't push yourself by trying to make it 2 to 3 hours. You may be so worn out that the next day you can't even take any weight. Your weeklong efforts may be in vain due to a single mistake. Don't forget that you could also injure yourself by pushing it so hard all the time.

3. Specific

While setting up the goals, you must define, measure, and create concrete steps to know what it will look like, realizing them in the real world. Also, plan for the next step as you gain momentum after a goal is achieved. It will help you to see where you were and where you are going.

Example: You should have decided to keep a journal as a part of your weight loss journey, and you are willing to have a firm grip over emotional eating. But, then, you should be considering some slight but significant behavioral changes. For example, make some time in addition to your regular writing hours; and, be prepared to not eat anything (even snack) after a meal. Create a time interval and process an evaluation through the new journal to see how it's going.

4. Time-limited

Scheduling is must while setting up goals. You can't just set up goals and wait for them to happen forever. Eventually, they will get lost in your daily hubbub and soon you will lose all energy and integrity to be in the game anymore. If the goal you have decided to take on takes a long time to be implemented, you can set some short or medium range goals for the time being. This will allow you to reach your ultimate goal. In addition, that will keep you focused without making you feel the long term goal is so incredibly difficult.

For example, if you are willing to get rid of all that extra fat in a year's time, then there should be some intermediate goals that would work as checkpoints indicating you are making real progress. Doing an inconsistent job won't help as they wouldn't bring any significance to your plan.

5. Flexible

The main characteristic of a good goal is that it's flexible. The reason is nothing but everything in this world changes with time. So, having an adaptation capability is important. A decision or strategy also follows the same rule. It has to be flexible so that it can accommodate any new idea and still make sense.

For instance, situations that might adverse your dieting plan will continuously occur. For example, invitations, social gatherings, late lunch in a restaurant, etc. Or the situation could be that you desperately want to break the routine for a day. Along with your goals, some contingency plans should be included to avoid situations like all-or-nothing that may enforce you to abandon your whole plan.

6. Be positive

Goals should be designed in such a way that they always seem positive rather than a burden. Psychologist have found that human beings do their best when they are trying to accomplish something as opposed to when they are attempting to avoid something.

For instance, a big part of weight loss ambition is avoiding lucrative junk foods that are low in nutrition. This is common that people put their goals as words in a notebook. Try writing it down as "I'm going to increase the amount of calorie intake from healthy and nutritious food items." It is much better than writing: "I'm going to give up eating cheeseburgers!"

If you continue this for a few weeks, your brain will be able to forget the usual association between treat and chocolate. Using this method, set up the treat trigger by replacing chocolates with yogurt and lucrative fruits.

The last thing to know is that meeting goals are almost 90% dependent on an individual's behavior. No living being can claim he or she is flawless. So, you cannot always expect what you set up to take place. The idea of building some stress management plans and tools would be a great help in staying motivated without getting deviated from the original plan.

HANDLING TEMPTATION

Almost nothing could be tougher for a person than improving his or her eating habits, even if the situation is that he or she is doing their own cooking and shopping. But what if people around you, are not supportive and keep offering you foods every time they encounter you? For this reason, a collection of 13 typical situations has been compiled here, which also include escape routes to get out of such circumstances. Regardless of their differences, the basic premise of each situation is: Be prepared. When you have a backup plan or a script of what to say in such situations, maintaining your changed eating habit shouldn't be interrupted. Let's look at some examples:

One of your colleagues is having a birthday party at work: Refusing a piece from your colleague's birthday cake means almost the same as refusing to sing "Happy Birthday!" You don't want to seem unsocial to others and you are not willing to breaking your newly achieved sacred foodie codes. You don't have to refuse the cake, just ask for a thinner slice. Then take an even smaller bite from the piece and leave out the icing and extra creams; just eat the cake. Office parties also entertain with sodas. Don't touch them. Instead, you can hold the coffee mug.

Your best pal asking for an ice cream break: Remember the days when you and your best friend used to spend hours in an ice cream cafe. You don't need to stop those outings entirely. What you need to change is your eating habit. Take a sorbet or frozen yogurt instead of ice creams that are rich in high calories.

Feeling desperately thirsty for a beer: When you're spending a vacation at the beach or working on a rough day in your workshop, looking for a beer is not uncommon. Grab a can, there's no harm in it. Just make sure it's a light brew. Pabst makes a particular version of low alcohol beer only containing 67 calories. Or, if you are more into old Miller Lite, go for it.

Only a few minutes left before a meal: You have got out of office and there's not enough time to sit down for an organized meal. The only option left may be fast-food, but you are avoiding it entirely, considering it untouchable. But you can still leave some menus open for your consumption as long as they are under a certain calorie level. You can even have meat sometimes as long as they are without the word 'crispy'.

Friends asking you to come to Starbucks: Most of the people who are on a diet program will look at you differently if you talk about Starbucks. It is like some kind of taboo. Avoid snacks that level up the amount of calories in your body. However, Starbucks is trying to develop their image and they are intending to welcome everyone to their shops, so they are offering menu items like Panini's and roll-ups. When it comes to drinks, pick anything with the name 'Skinny'—this will help you to cut the calorie count at least by a third.

When you are at a restaurant with your date: When you are visiting a special place with your date, you can get the meal square back at a reasonable calorie level. All you need to do is skip sauces or other additional ingredients. Additionally, there are many family restaurants that offer low-calorie meals. Thinking about dieting while eating is not feasible. Instead, you should consider ordering less food that are enriched with flavors. At first grab a little appetizer and share the others with your partner—is it not great to share food with your partner to enlighten the mood? Do the same for salads and soups. If you are going to have dessert afterward, it is fine, but make sure you order with the one with mostly fruits and don't forget to share it.

Your partner gifts you a box of chocolate: At first you need to know a quick lesson. Your lover doesn't intend for the chocolates to be eaten instantly, you may always take a smaller piece and taste it, take your time and share.

You went shopping while feeling hungry: Lengthy shopping is like a marathon - both taking a constant high energy level. Avoid spending all your time sitting in the food court of the mall. Rather take some roasted nuts and a hot pretzel. A pretzel should not count for more than 490 calories with only 8 grams of saturated fat. With a minimal amount of 2 grams of fiber and one gram saturated fat, it's a good choice, especially when you plan to eat over time.

You have got to catch the early morning flight: There cannot be a better option than a Starbucks in an airport. Soy milk with venti latte is more than what you could wish for breakfast. Also, add a refreshing shot of espresso that would give you 170 calories in total. To save yourself from the trouble of standing in a long queue of other people waiting to get breakfast, let's get started with a yogurt and banana. They are less than 400 calories, and you see a start to your day in just ten minutes.

In a picnic there's nothing left except hot dogs and hamburgers: At most BBQ parties, people get trapped by the scenic outdoors. The good news is, meat grills are found to be much less fatty than pan fried. Unfortunately, most grillers tend to rely on dogs and greasy burgers to feed everyone without any extra labor. On the other hand, traditional slaws and potato salads remain stuffed with calories. But the worst is that it is hard to resist the fragrance of wafting smoke. Not a problem: go ahead and try to smell the burgers as much as you can but don't eat them, eat the hot dog. A hot dog with bun and covered with sauce should push the calorie level to 250 calories. This equates the calorie counting in a burger's fat alone! Burger fixings are welcome, but you have got to use fixings like tomato, onion, and lettuce.

It's almost 3:30 pm and you're feeling the hungry beast inside: Some natural factors are responsible in the first place for a drop in energy level. Primarily: mild dehydration, lack of iron in the body, light lunch, and the crash of the coffee taken late morning. Before starting your journey toward the cafeteria, get a big glass of water in hand. The water consumption will make you feel full and as a side result it will boost your blood flow. To eradicate all those cobwebs formed as a result of restlessness from the morning, have a cup of coffee with iron-rich cinnamon.

While drinking with co-workers: Soda, fruit juices, and any other kind of mixes increase the level of calories in cocktails. So, when you hit the bar to celebrate your colleague or friend's promotion why not toast with a low-calorie cocktail? Clear liquors with soda and lime offer the most bang for your buck.

Your beloved family members try to make you eat what they want: When your mom wants you to try her new recipe, they also try to make you full in the process. In other words, it's a reflection of love. And as you praise her cooking, she will fill your plate with more of that newly cooked stuff! What do you do now?! Instead of sitting in front of the plate all the time, help your parents with clean up and serving. In this way, you can be assured that you are out of their radar. Additionally, your parents get that feeling that they have raised a caring child.

CONCLUSION

I want to personally thank you again for reading this book!

I sincerely hope the information presented will help you to understand the benefits of the HCG Diet. Moreover, the resume of clinical studies on the last chapter should clear any doubts in your mind regarding the safety and efficacy of the hCG diet as long as your diet regimen religiously adheres to the calorie restriction and recommended food selection. It is of paramount significance that your hCG dosage determination and injections be performed by duly trained physicians in the protocol.

I hope that you feel ready to take action and finally lose those unwanted pounds using the resources discussed. The next step is to put into practice the methods and employ the strategies we've discussed here to begin losing that weight for good! It's safe and easy.

Finally, if you enjoyed this book, please take the time to share your thoughts and post a positive review on Amazon. I would greatly appreciate your support!

Thank you and good luck!

Benjamin Tideas

COPYRIGHT NOTICE

ADDITIONAL RESOURCES

Please point your web browser to
http://www.plaid-enterprises.com/hcg
for more resources, my full bibliography and to grab your FREE book!

Finally, I hope you enjoy the recipes that follow!

BONUS: HCG DIET RECIPES

Following are just a few recipes, adapted from many sources, for every part of your day that will help you vary your food choices, but still stick to the HCG Diet. Enjoy!!

BROCCOLI & FETA OMELET WITH TOAST

Preparation Time: 5 minutes
Cooking Time: 10 minutes
Yield: 1 serving (1 omelet and 2 pieces toast)

Ingredients

Cooking spray
1 broccoli one cup (chopped)
2 eggs (large)
2 tbsp feta cheese, crumbled
1/4 teaspoon dill (dried)
2 slices of toasted rye bread

Preparation

Take a nonstick skillet and heat it over medium heat. Use the cooking spray to coat the pan and then add broccoli. Cook it for three minutes. Mix dill, egg, and feta in a bowl. Pour down the eggs in the pan and cook it for about 4 minutes; flip the omelet and keep cooking for another 2 minutes. When done, serve with toast.

SPICED GREEN TEA SMOOTHIE

Preparation Time: 30 minutes
Cooking Time: 5 minutes
Yields: Makes 2 servings (serving size: 1 cup)

Ingredients

3/4 cup strong chilled green tea
1/8 tbsp cayenne pepper
2-3 tbsp lemon juice
2 tbsp agave nectar
1 small pear, cut into pieces with skin on
2 tbsp plain yogurt (fat-free)
7-8 ice cubes

Preparation

Put everything in a blender and process until it becomes smooth. Drink cold.

CHOCOLATE-DIPPED BANANA BITES

Ingredients

2 tbsp chocolate chips (semisweet)
1 small banana cut into one-inch chunks

Preparation

At first take the chocolate chips in a small microwave bowl. To melt the chocolates microwave it at high until it melts. Put banana pieces in chocolate.

BANANA & ALMOND BUTTER TOAST

Preparation Time: 5 minutes
Total Time required: 5 minutes
Yield: 1 serving

Ingredients

1 tbsp almond butter
1 slice toasted rye bread
1 sliced banana

Preparation

On toast spread the almond butter. Complete the topping with banana slices.

HONEY GRAPEFRUIT WITH BANANA

Prep: 5 minutes. This is the perfect meal for breakfast, especially when you are super hungry.

Ingredients

1 (about 24-ounce) jar refrigerated red grapefruit
1 cup banana (sliced)
1 tbsp fresh chopped mint
1 tbsp honey

Preparation

Reserve 1/4 cup juice and drain grapefruit sections.
Put juice, grapefruit sections, and any other ingredients in a medium sized bowl. Toss the bowl gently to coat. It's now ready to Serve immediately.

WHITE BEAN WITH HUMMUS AND CRUDITES

Preparation Time: 5 minutes
Yield: 1 serving

Ingredients

Quarter cup drained and rinsed canned white beans
1 tbsp chopped chives
1 tbsp lemon juice
2 tbsp olive oil
Raw vegetables (assorted) such as chopped broccoli florets, sliced green and red peppers and carrots.

Preparation

1. Combine chives, lemon juice, beans, and oil in a small bowl. Mash them all with a fork to make them smooth.

2. Serve with raw vegetables (half cup) like carrots, sugar snap peas, cucumbers, broccoli, grape tomatoes, and bell peppers.

BBQ TURKEY BURGERS

Yield: Burgers for 4 people

Ingredients

1 pound meat turkey
1 minced garlic clove
1/2 tbsp paprika
1/4 teaspoon cumin
Pinch of salt (kosher)
Quarter teaspoon freshly ground black pepper
4 slices grilled sweet onion
Quarter cup barbecue sauce
4 (1.6-oz) toasted sesame seed buns

Preparation

1. In a medium size bowl mix turkey, garlic, paprika, and cumin.
2. Form turkey into 4 patties; season with pepper and salt.
3. Heat grill to medium-high and cook each side (turn after 7 minutes each) and then serve with desired buns and topping.

MIDDLE EASTERN RICE SALAD

Ingredients

2 tbsp olive oil
½ thinly sliced sweet onion
1 can rinsed and drained chickpeas
1/2 teaspoon ground cumin
1/4 teaspoon salt
Freshly ground black pepper
Three cups of cooked brown rice
1/2 cup chopped pitted dates
1/4 cup chopped mint
1/4 cup chopped parsley

Preparation

1. Take a nonstick skillet to heat the oil over medium. Cook and stir after adding onions until they get brown. Stop heating and stir in chickpeas, salt and cumin; season to taste with ground black pepper.
2. Combine mint rice, onion-chickpea mixture, parsley, and dates in a big bowl; toss them altogether thoroughly. Serve either at warm or at room temperature.

ENERGY-REVVING QUINOA

Ingredients

1 cup cooked quinoa
1/3 cup canned low-sodium black beans, drained and rinsed
1 small tomato, chopped
1 scallion, sliced
1 teaspoon olive oil
1 teaspoon fresh lemon juice
Pinch of salt
Pinch of freshly ground black pepper

Preparation

Take a medium bowl and toss everything together.

BREAKFAST BARLEY WITH BANANA & SUNFLOWER SEEDS

Preparation Time: 5 minutes
Cooking Time: 10 minutes
Yield: 1 person

Ingredients

2/3 cup water
1/3 cup quick-cooking pearl barley (uncooked)
1 sliced banana
1 tbsp unsalted salted sunflower seeds
1 teaspoon honey

Preparation

1. Mix 2/3 cup water and barley in a microwave bowl and microwave on HIGH 6 minutes.
2. Stir and let stand 2 minutes.
3. Make topping with banana slices, sunflower seeds and honey

CURRIED EGG SALAD SANDWHICH

Preparation Time: 5 minutes
Yield: 1 sandwich

Ingredients

2 chopped hard-cooked eggs,
2 tbsp plain Greek-style yogurt
2 tbsp chopped red bell pepper
1/4 teaspoon curry powder
1/8 teaspoon salt
1/8 teaspoon pepper
2 slices toasted rye bread
1/2 cup spinach
1 orange

Preparation

1. Combine yogurt, eggs, curry powder, bell pepper, pepper, and, salt in a small bowl and then stir well.
2. Place spinach on rye bread, serve the orange on the side and top with egg salad.

SALMON NOODLE BOWL

Preparation Time: 8 minutes
Cooking Time: 20 mins.
Yield: Makes 2 servings

Ingredients

4 ounces soba buckwheat noodles
5 ounces asparagus
Cooking spray
1 Salmon fillet, skin off, cut into eight pieces
1 tablespoon toasted sesame oil
Zest and juice of 1-2 limes
Quarter teaspoon kosher salt
Quarter tsp pepper
4 ounces cucumber, skin on, cut into medium pieces
Half avocado (cut into bite-size pieces)

Preparation

1. Boil the noodles until soft. Transfer with tongs to a strainer. Add the asparagus to same boiling water. Cook until for 2 minutes; rinse under water (cold).
2. Heat a grill pan or skillet over medium-high heat. Cook the salmon until cooked through; cook it for three minutes per side.
3. Make the vinaigrette: Mix together lime zest, sesame oil, juice, and salt and pepper - everything in a little bowl. Mix the asparagus, noodles, and vinaigrette in a medium size bowl.
4. Add the cucumber and avocado; toss to coat. Just before serving, add salmon. Serve warm or at room temperature, or refrigerate 4 hours.

GREEK YOGURT GRUIT PARFAIT

Preparation Time: Five minutes
Yield: Makes 1 serving

Ingredients

3/4 cup fat-free Greek yogurt
2 cups sliced mixed plums, nectarines, and peaches
3/4 cup rice cereal (puffed)
2 tbsp walnuts and almonds (toasted and chopped)
1 tbsp ground flaxseed
1 tbsp maple syrup, agave nectar, or honey

Preparation

In a tall 4-cup container or jar, layer half of the yogurt cereal, flaxseed, nuts, and some syrup. Do the same as well with the remaining half of ingredients; last of all add syrup. Keep it in fridge for about 5 hours.

BLACK BEAN AND CHICKEN CHILAQUILES

Ingredients

Cooking spray
1 cup onion (sliced)
5 garlic minced cloves
2 cups cooked chicken breast (shredded)
1 can rinsed and drained black beans
1 cup fatless, low-sodium chicken broth
1 (3/4-ounce) can salsa fresco
15 tortillas (1 inch strip each)
1 cup quesoblanco (shredded)

Preparation

Preheat oven to 450°.

Heat a nonstick skillet with keeping the temperature over medium-high. Use cooking spray to coat pan. Now use the onions: sauté 5 minutes or until browned. Now add garlic and sauté for 1 minute. Add the pieces of chicken; cook for half minute. Now take a medium bowl to put the mixtures and stir in beans. At last add broth and salsa to pan. Wait sometimes to boil. Gradually decrease heat and simmer five minutes, while stirring.

Place 1/2 of tortilla strips in the bottom of an eleven by seven inch baking dish coated with cooking spray. Layer the remaining chicken mixtures over tortillas and top with the rest of tortillas and chicken mixture. Now pour the mixture (broth) evenly, gently over chicken mixture. Sprinkle it with something like cheese. Now it would need just 10 minutes on top at 450 degrees to melt the cheese and get that brownish look.

SPICY SOUTHWESTERN BLACK BEAN CHILI

Preparation Time: 15 minutes
Cooking Time: Ten minutes
Yield: Makes for persons

Ingredients

2 teaspoons oil (olive)
1 large onion (chopped)
1 cup (seeded and chopped) jalapeno
1 finely chopped large garlic clove
2 tbsp chili powder
1 teaspoon ground cumin
4 boxes of tomato soup and roasted red pepper
2 cans rinsed and drained black beans
Quarter cup reduced-fat sour cream
Quarter cup fresh cilantro (chopped)
Half cup firm-ripe diced peeled avocado Cilantro sprigs (optional)

Preparation

Take a medium saucepan heat the oil at medium temperature. Now add some onion and jalapeño; cook and stir until they soften (about three minutes). Stir in the garlic, and cumin, chili powder; cook for one minute. Again stir in black beans and soup. Simmer for five minutes. Now, put in the cilantro (chopped). Ladle the soup into a bowl and then top with one tbsp of sour cream, cilantro sprigs, and avocado.

CREAMY AVOCADO CUPS

Ingredients

1 avocado
1 tbsp lime juice
1 tbsp reduced-fat sour cream or plain yogurt
Quarter teaspoon ground cumin
1 tbsp fresh cilantro (chopped)
12 endive leaves

Preparation

Pit, Peel, and one mashed avocado and set aside. Combine 1 tbsp lime juice, 1 tbsp reduced-fat sour cream or yogurt, quarter teaspoon ground cumin, and 1 tbsp chopped fresh cilantro in a small sized bowl. Now stir in avocado. Start spooning avocado mixture gradually and evenly into 12 endive leaves.

PAN-GRILLED SALMON WITH PINEAPPLE SALSA

Ingredients

1 cup fresh pineapple (chopped)
2 tbsp finely chopped red onion
2 tbsp chopped cilantro
1 tbsp rice vinegar
1/8 teaspoon ground red pepper
Cooking spray
4 Salmon fillets (1/2 inch thick each)
Half teaspoon salt

Preparation

Mix first five ingredients in a medium bowl and set aside.

Coat the grill pan with cooking spray. Heat it over medium-high heat. Sprinkle the fishes with salt. Cook fish for four minutes on each side or until it flakes easily when it is tested with a fork. Prepare topping with salsa.

ITALIAN GARBANZO SALAD

Ingredients

3 cups finely chopped fennel bulb
2 cups chopped tomato
1 cup chopped red onion
1 cup fresh basil (chopped)
1/3 cup balsamic vinegar
1 tbsp olive oil
1 teaspoon freshly ground black pepper
Quarter teaspoon salt
4 minced garlic cloves
2 cans of rinsed and drained chickpeas (garbanzo beans),
Half cup crumbled feta cheese

Preparation

Mix all ingredients but leave out the cheese in a bowl; now toss very well. Wait for half an hour and sprinkle with cheese afterward.

RAW KALE, GRAPEFRUIT AND TOASTED HAZELNUT SALAD

Preparation Time: Fifteen minutes
Yield: Makes for 4 persons

Ingredients

2 grapefruit
Half small red onion, thinly sliced and divided
Quarter cup fresh lemon juice
Half cup fat-free plain yogurt
2 tbsp extra-virgin olive oil
Half teaspoon kosher salt
1/4 teaspoon black pepper
8 ounces lacinato kale (thinly sliced), or baby kale leaves
1 ounce toasted hazelnuts (chopped)

Preparation

1. First of all, segment and peel the grapefruits; keep 3 tablespoons juice in a big bowl. Mince 2 rings onion, and combine with grapefruit juice, with salt, oil, yogurt, pepper, and lemon juice. Whisk them all until well mixed.
2. Toss in a kale. Top with remaining and hazelnuts, onion, and grapefruit.

DARK CHOCOLATE & OAT CLUSTERS

Preparation Time: 5 minutes
Cooking Time: 3 minutes
Total Time: Ten minutes
Yield: 4 servings

Ingredients

2 tbsp peanut butter
2 tbsp 1% low-fat milk
Quarter cup semisweet chocolate chips
3/4 cup rolled oats (old-fashioned)

Preparation

1. Heat chocolate chips, milk, and peanut butter in a saucepan over low heat for three minutes or until chips melt.
2. Stir in oats before removing from heat.
3. With a spoon or small ice cream scoop drop eight ball-shaped portions on a wax paper—lined baking sheet. Keep it in a fridge for ten minutes.

AVOCADO WHIP

Preparation Time: 5 minutes
Yield: Makes 2 cups (serving size: quarter cup)

Ingredients

2 avocados (pitted and peeled)
Quarter cup fresh lime juice (about 3 limes)
1 tbsp tahini
Quarter cup chopped onion
Quarter teaspoon kosher salt
Quarter teaspoon fresh pepper

Preparation

Put everything in a food processor, now process for thirty seconds. Transfer the mix to a serving dish. Now, set aside 1 tablespoon lime juice, drizzle it over the surface, and cover with plastic wrap and refrigerate. Finally, garnish with pepper.

CRISP CHICKENPEA SLAW

Preparation Time: 10 minutes
Yield: Makes 2 servings (serving size: 3 half cup)

Ingredients

Quarter cup fat-free plain yogurt
1 tbsp cider vinegar
1 tbsp water
Quarter teaspoon kosher salt
Freshly ground black pepper
1 (15-oz) can rinsed and drained low-sodium chickpeas
2 cups packed green cabbage (sliced)
2 thinly sliced stalks celery
2 carrots, peeled and thinly sliced, or two cups shredded carrots
2 tbsp toasted sesame seeds

Preparation

Take a medium size bowl; stir together the vinegar, yogurt, salt, pepper, and water to taste. Add the celery, chickpeas, carrots, and carrots; toss them altogether to combine. Finally, sprinkle with sesame seeds.
Transfer slaw to portable containers. Cool down in refrigerator for 4 hours before serving.

RED-LENTIL HUMMUS

Preparation Time: 5 minutes
Cooking Time: 25 minutes
Yield: Makes: 3 cups

Ingredients

1 cup red lentils, rinsed
Half teaspoon sea salt, plus more for finishing
Quarter cup tahini
Half garlic clove, smashed
3 tbsp olive oil
Juice of half lemon
1 teaspoon red-wine vinegar
Quarter teaspoon coriander
1 tbsp extra-virgin olive oil for drizzling
Pinch sweet paprika
Half tablespoons minced parsley
Greek yogurt

Preparation

1. Place lentils in a 2-quarter pot and cover with two cups water. First Boil, and then reduce heat, and simmer for 20 minutes to tender.
2. Combine salt, tahini, lentils, olive oil, garlic, vinegar, coriander, and lemon juice in a food processor and blend until smooth.
3. Before serving: Spoon hummus into a deep bowl. Drizzle over with olive oil. Now, sprinkle with parsley and paprika.

BANANA NUT OATMEAL

Preparation Time: 5 minutes
Cooking Time: 5 minutes
Yield: 1 serving (1 1/2 cups)

Ingredients

Half cup old-fashioned rolled oats
1 cup water
1 banana (sliced)
1 tbsp chopped walnuts
1 teaspoon cinnamon

Preparation

Mix oats and one cup water in a small microwave-safe bowl and microwave on high three minutes.
Top with cinnamon, walnuts, banana slices.

GREEK LENTIL SOUP WITH TOASTED PITA

Preparation Time: 10 minutes
Cooking Time: 20 minutes
Yield: Four people

Ingredients

1 tbsp olive oil
2 celery stalks, chopped
2 carrots, peeled and chopped
1 onion
2 minced garlic cloves
2 teaspoons dried oregano
Half teaspoon salt
Half teaspoon pepper
8 cups water
1 cup dry lentils
2 tbsp fresh lemon juice (about 1 lemon)
4 whole-grain pitas, each cut into 4 triangles and toasted

Preparation

1. Use a Dutch oven to heat the oil at medium; add carrot, celery, garlic, oregano, onion, pepper and salt; cook for five minutes.
2. Add the water and lentils. Simmer, and keep it partially covered for about fifteen minutes.
3. Use a hand blender or potato masher to puree the soup until semi-smooth and thick.
4. Drizzle with lemon juice; serve with toasted pita triangles.

HAM, SLICED PEAR AND SWISS SANDWHICH

Preparation Time: 5 minutes
Yield: One Serving

Ingredients

1 tbsp plain Greek-style low-fat yogurt
Quarter teaspoon dried dill
2 slices pumpernickel bread
1 ounce lean sliced ham
1 small pear, thinly sliced
1 1- ounce slice Swiss cheese

Preparation

Mix dill and yogurt a small bowl, stir until blended.
Spread the yogurt mix on bread slices. Top with 1 bread slice with ham, 1/2 of pear slices, remaining bread slice, and cheese. Use the remaining pear slices to serve.

SUNFLOWER LENTIL SPREAD

Ingredients

1 canned lentils, rinsed and drained
1 tbsp lemon juice
Quarter teaspoon salt
Quarter teaspoon pepper
2 tbsp sunflower seeds
1 finely diced celery stalk
1 finely diced scallion
2 tbsp chopped fresh parsley
2 halved pitas

Preparation

1. Mix, lemon juice, salt, lentils, and pepper in a blender; blend until smooth.
2. Stir in sunflower celery, scallions, seeds, and parsley.
3. Microwave pita at high temperature for one minute and then serve with spread.

SPICED BANANA-ALMOND SMOOTHIE

Ingredients

1 banana (ripe)
1 cup almond milk (unsweetened)
1 tbsp almond butter
Half teaspoon ground cardamom
1 tbsp honey
2 ice cubes

Preparation

Combine all the ingredients and put them in a blender. Blend them until smooth.

EGG AND RICE SALAD TO GO

Ingredients

Half cup brown rice (cooked)
1 cup roughly chopped cooked green beans
1 ripe plum (thinly sliced)
2 tbsp chopped walnuts
1 hard-cooked egg (sliced)
1 teaspoon sesame oil
2 tbsp fresh lime juice
Quarter teaspoon kosher salt
Freshly ground black pepper

Preparation

Mix beans, walnuts, rice, egg, and plum in a carriable container.
Drizzle with pepper, lime juice, sesame oil, and salt and toss gently to mix. Refrigerate for two days.

And some final quickies!

Peanut Butter and Fruit with Bagel
Ingredients
1 Thomas' 100% Whole Wheat Bagel Thin
2 tbsp peanut butter
1 medium banana (sliced)
4 strawberries (sliced)
Total: 430 calories

☐

Egg & Cheese Breakfast Bowl
This breakfast bowl takes cheese, egg whites, turkey, sausage, and potatoes into a protein-packed morning meal.

Microwave a Jimmy Dean D-Lights Breakfast Bowl and pair it with one slice whole wheat toast. Finally, use 6 oz. orange juice to wash it down.

Total calories: 380

☐

Peanut Butter Soy Smoothie
At first, blend 1 cup vanilla soy milk, half banana, 1 tbsp peanut butter, Quarter tsp cinnamon, and finally, six ice cubes.

Take a toasted English muffin and pair with it; don't forget to spread 2 tsp fruit jam over the toast.

Total calories: 390

☐

Blueberry Nut Oatmeal
Cook half cup dry Quick one-minute Quaker Oats
Top with one cup frozen blueberries, and 1 tbsp honey, and 2 tbsp cashews
Total calories: 390

☐

Superfast Chef Salad
To make the salad, combine two cups salad greens with 2 ounces of water-packed drained canned tuna and quarter cup cooked chickpeas. Top with 2 tablespoon reduced-fat cheese (shredded) and two tbsp fat-free ranch dressing.

Take a dinner Rolland pair with it.

Total calories: 408

☐

Barbecue Chicken Pita
Stir together 1 tablespoon BBQ sauce and half cup chopped precooked chicken. And then microwave for thirty seconds.

Cut a whole wheat pita in half; then, inside push the chicken mix.

Use 1 cup chopped lettuce to top, 2 tablespoon diced cucumber and 1 tablespoon fat-free ranch dressing.

Use ten baby carrots to pair.

Total calories: 405

www.ingramcontent.com/pod-product-compliance
Lightning Source LLC
Chambersburg PA
CBHW070611290526
45790CB00002B/873